Oil Pulling

The Magic of Ancient Era

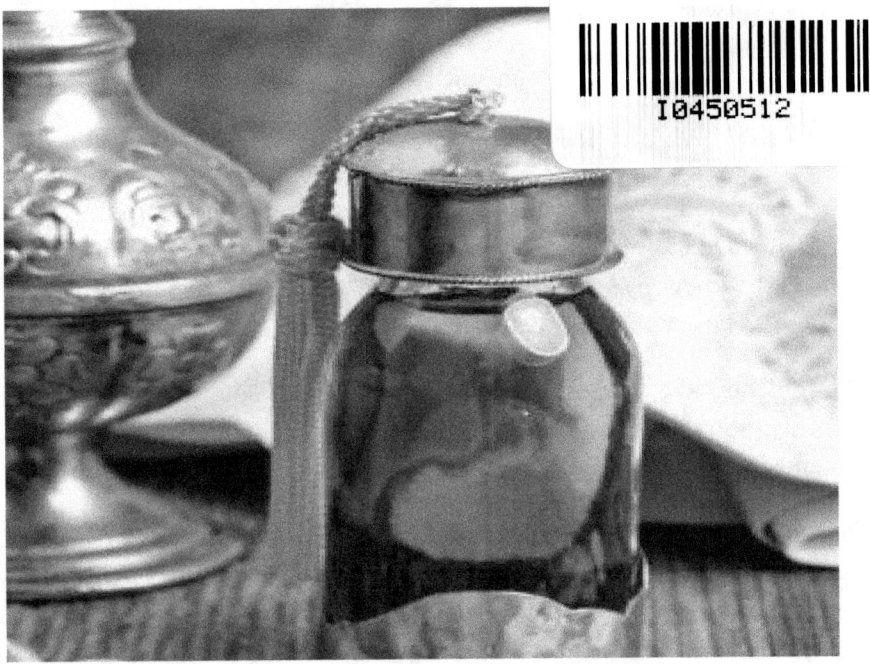

Health Learning Series

M. Usman

Mendon Cottage Books

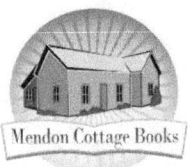

JD-Biz Publishing

Disclaimer

The information is this book is provided for informational purposes only. It is not intended to be used and medical advice or a substitute for proper medical treatment by a qualified health care provider. The information is believed to be accurate as presented based on research by the author.

The contents have not been evaluated by the U.S. Food and Drug Administration or any other Government or Health Organization and the contents in this book are not to be used to treat cure or prevent disease.

The author or publisher is not responsible for the use or safety of any diet, procedure or treatment mentioned in this book. The author or publisher is not responsible for errors or omissions that may exist.

Warning

The Book is for informational purposes only and before taking on any diet, treatment or medical procedure, it is recommended to consult with your primary health care provider.

Our books are available at

1. Amazon.com
2. Barnes and Noble
3. Itunes
4. Kobo
5. Smashwords
6. Google Play Books

Table of Contents

Preface

Oil pulling, the magical phenomenon, is still a mystery for the masses. In this book we shall try to unveil the things behind this ayurvedic technique, which will make your oral healthcare easier.

Oil pulling is an ancient phenomenon revisited in the early twentieth century by Dr. Karach. We have tried to provide you with all the oil pulling questions that befuddle you. We have started off with a history and the background for you so that you can come to terms with this non-medical medicine for your mouth. Once you are familiar with its roots, we explain the precise methodology, using several references of various sites and amalgamating the accurate ones.

Oil pulling has several benefits, as you will come to know, but what is important to understand is that oil pulling is not a magic potion that will heal everything. Basically, as emphasized by several doctors, our mouth is the main source for the entrance of germs and diseases and what oil pulling solely helps in doing is to keep our mouths bacteria free. However, the benefits outweigh the problems, as you will find that there are no side effects to this natural technique and all it need is your time and regularity.

We will also go through the diseases that these bad bacteria spread in an unclean mouth so that you can see how serious the complete picture actually is and how crucial the cleanliness of your mouth is.

We conclude by giving you multiple oil using options and their benefits and our final opinion on oil pulling, the magical technique.

Chapter 1: Introduction

Oil pulling therapy probably raises a lot of questions as your mind starts to imagine all sorts of interpretations instantaneously, doesn't it? Well don't worry; we have the answers to the questions your brain is boggling you with. Let's have a basic introduction to what is oil pulling.

Oil pulling is also termed as oil swishing. It is an ancient technique that is simple, cost effective, and a purely natural remedy for oral and systematic health benefits. It is taken from the ayurvedic text Charaka Samhita, in which it is termed as "Kaval Gandusha" or "Kavala Graha". It is known to cure around thirty systematic diseases from headaches and migraines to diabetes and asthma. The methodology of oil pulling is extremely simple as we will discuss it in our second section, but it instills confusion in the minds of the general population as it is from an ancient text and has gone through several interpretations. We aim to clarify all the misconceptions and enlighten you with this natural remedy technique.

We plan to walk you through the entire process; its background, methodology, how to properly make use of it and the benefits we reap from this natural technique. Let us begin by analyzing the initiation of this technique and its roots to give you a complete picture for a more comprehensive understanding.

1.1 Background

Understanding something completely requires a study of its roots and in the case of the oil pulling technique, it means the understanding of how Ayurveda works. Ayurveda is derived from the Sanskrit words "Ayur" and "Veda". Ayur means longevity and Veda means knowledge. Thus this gives us the purpose of the meaning, and the knowledge that helps in achieving longevity. This comes from the self-realization aspect and is the ultimate goal of life for every individual. Yoga and Ayurveda aim at the harmonization of the physical body so that our inner consciousness can come under action as well.

The medication base of this technique comes from the Samkhya philosophy and it means to know the truth. It was believed that each individual's constitution and personality is determined by the combination of three doshas that remain unchanged throughout our lifetime and are as individual to each as the finger prints. These doshas are of motion, metabolism and cohesiveness of the body. They are different for each individual, as everyone has a difference in their metabolism, motions and cohesiveness. The equilibrium of the three doshas is believed to be important for optimal health.

The literature on oil pulling therapies is taken from the Charaka Samihta, which was written in around 1500BC. It has classified more than 200 diseases and 150 pathological conditions and inherited defects and all of them were remarkably in consistence with WHO disease classification criteria. Ayurveda laid the foundations for the emphasis on repeated observations and acceptance of the data, only in the case of uniform consistency.

1.2 Recent Resurfacing

Oil pulling, and the current usage, was popularized in 1990s by one of the old adopters' Lt. Col Tummala Koteswara Rao from Bangalore, India. Rao actively practiced and promoted this technique in India along with other ayurvedic processes. The articles by Rao were published in English and several other native languages all over the nation.

Rao came into the revelation of this process through the paper of Dr. Karach, in which he introduced and revised the technique by emphasizing on swishing and not gargling in the mouth, and the usage of vegetable oil for this process. The paper was very successful and was circulated in German magazines as well. This focus in the early 1990s brought this process into the light of many, and several people began to take it seriously. However, the misconceptions reigned and confusion clouded the masses from adopting it on a daily basis.

Chapter 2: The Optimum Methodology

The initial condition is that oil pulling has to be performed first thing in the morning. It has to be performed with an empty stomach and even drinking water has to be avoided.

Step 1: Pour exactly 1 tablespoon of sunflower or sesame oil (or any other oil, for instance, coconut oil can be chosen). Children are only to be allowed to perform this if they have the practice to avoid swallowing any amounts of oil. You can also use lesser quantity of oil for them.

Step 2: Swirl the oil in your mouth properly, and be careful to avoid swallowing. Move it around your mouth through your teeth as you do with your mouthwash. Avoid gargles though, as that would lead to you swallowing and the purpose is not to include the throat in it. The oil will start to get watery as your saliva combines with it. Relax your mouth and do not put too much oil as that will make your jaw sore. The purpose is to achieve comfort, use your tongue to help in the swirling process.

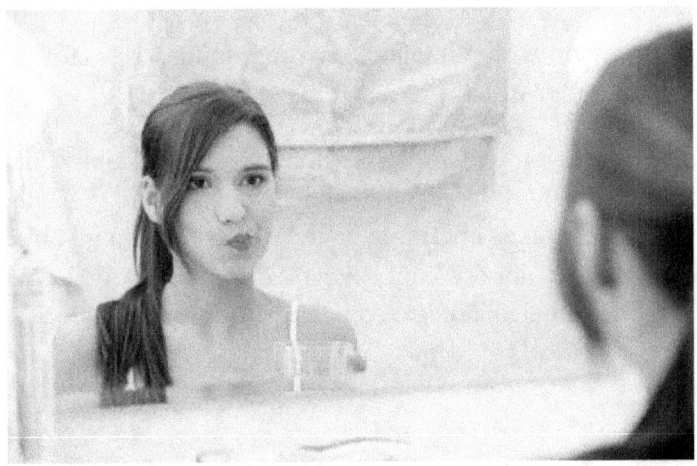

Remember, do not get too conscious. This is not a very technical process and do not over think it, rather, be natural in your performance. Be gentle in swirling and continue for around twenty minutes. You can throw it out earlier if it becomes too unpleasant or you have an unbearable urge to swallow it. Initial reactions of people are that it is a little unpleasant but don't worry as you will get used to its taste, like brushing your teeth. The time of twenty minutes is just a rule of thumb; it may vary with the type of oil used. The point of indication is that when the oil has absorbed the toxins it turns whitish and gets thinner. So if you spit it earlier you may do this again as the process will not have served its purpose.

Step 3: The last step. Spit out the oil and rinse your mouth with warm salt water. It is not necessary but it is helpful in soothing any inflammation and can also be effective in rinsing out any leftover toxins in the mouth. You may repeat this process daily or several times a week. Use breaks in between, as there is no fixed frequency and each can make up their own routine. One immediate benefit is whiter teeth and a cleaner mouth and believe me that is just the start of the benefits.

2.1 Important Notes to Methodology

➢ This process has to be done only in the mornings, unless absolutely necessary. Perform this method three to four hours after the intake of food and the timings depend upon the food you have consumed.

➢ Do not brush before oil pulling, clean your mouth with warm water and salt after which you may brush.

➢ With experience you will notice the time the oil is turning white and the completion of the process will become clear to you. Keep noting the time it takes in turning white every time you go through this process. The color does not have to be completely white and close to white can also indicate completion of the process.

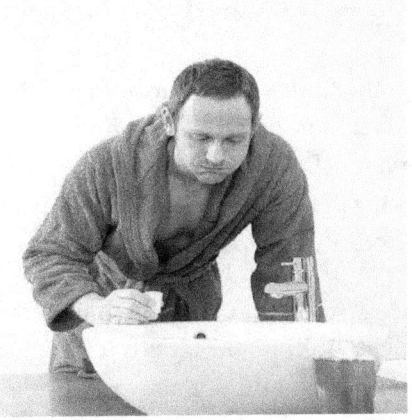

- ➢ A little swallowing is not harmful as the digestive system has the capability to eliminate these toxins, but if you feel the urge to swallow too much then spit the entire contents out.

- ➢ To make sure your toothbrush is toxin free, use a different one for after oil pulling and a separate one for using at night.

- ➢ There are no diet restrictions after completing the oil pulling process.

- ➢ Do not spit the contents of your mouth in the sink as they can clog your pipes with the passage of time. Throw them out in an empty trash can.

Chapter 3: Purpose and Effectiveness

Oil pulling removes the toxins from our body. Arsenic is an example of a toxin that we inhale through the air and food that we intake. Arsenic taken in organic form, like from out natural surroundings, isn't really harmful for the body but the inorganic arsenic obtained from food can have negative impacts on our body.

Oral healthcare is tended by this oil pulling measure that we adopt. The intense movement of oil in our mouth releases us from many chronic disorders, germs, and inflammatory foci that usually stick to the roots of our teeth. The roots of the teeth extend far into the jaw bone region and its cavities. When microbes enter the tooth neck they find the warm and damp conditions perfectly suitable for them and they establish themselves. This is known as dental foci and they damage the body through their metabolic products. They cause damage to the teeth and weaken your immune system and can have a weak effect on the internal organs of the body as well. The oil causes a marked mucosal and tissue perfusion and the vitamins in the oil are absorbed by the mucous membranes. The oil absorbs the toxins as well, thus removing them from your system.

3.1 Consequence of an Unhealthy Mouth

Acids cause the demineralization of teeth by leeching out contents, like calcium, from its tissues. These acids are produced by specific types of bacteria like lactobacilli and mutans streptococci. These are the makers' of the cavities in the mouth and consume and produce waste exactly like humans. The waste created is extremely acidic and helps the demineralization.

The primary food source for these bacteria is dietary sugars. This includes sucrose (table sugar), glucose, fructose, lactose and cooked starches.

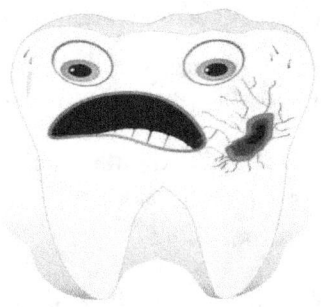

Remember that the foods you eat are the same food items that are available to the bacteria that live in your mouth. So, when you consume foods that contain sugars, they get a meal too. And within minutes they start producing the acids that cause tooth decay. Therefore it is wise that when you eat sugar products you finish them quickly. By doing this you can make sure that these food items do not remain for a long time in your mouth.

Inside our mouth is the place where the bacteria reside and the part that holds the acids is called dental plaque. The acids get accumulated underneath the plaque or get seeped out into the mouth. The acid that gets seeped out is not harmful since the saliva present in our mouth dilutes those acids immediately. However the acid that seeps through the plaque down to the surface of the tooth causes its demineralization. The dental plaque provides a cover for those harmful acids protecting them from getting diluted or being washed away. Saliva can finally travel down there and dilute the acids, but this process may take a couple of hours and the damage would already be inflicted.

That means that the acid will remain relatively concentrated for an extended period. During this whole time, tooth demineralization will take place. Hence, you can see that it is essential that you brush and floss but use oil pulling as well as it will help you in taking these acids out of the protection of the dental plaque and wash them out from your system.

The buildup of this dental plaque introduces us to another very serious problem, Gingivitis. Even if you brush your teeth, this plaque reforms fairly quickly within 24 hours. If these plaques remain in your mouth for more than a couple of days it forms tartar. Once its transformation takes place, the plaque is now even harder to brush away and will become an even friendlier environment for the bacteria. The process for its removal is now only with the dentist and he uses the scaling procedure to get rid of the tartar.

Now with the tartar being present in the mouth it begins to cause irritation in the gum sand causes them to get inflamed. The gums then get swollen and will likely start bleeding.

The gum disease that initiates can create a lot of problems for you; the following are a few examples:

- Weakened immune system

- Diabetes

- Hormonal changes

- Viral infections

- Stress

Let's have a look at the symptoms of this gum disease or more properly termed gingivitis:

- Painful or tender gums

- Signs of swelling in the gums

- Gums becoming softer

- Color of the gums turning from pink to dusky red

- Gums bleeding after brushing

Symptoms of a more severe stage of gingivitis

- Body temperatures rising

- General malaise

- Painful gums

- Excessive saliva production

- Metallic taste in the mouth

- Ulcers in between the teeth

3.2 Linking your mouth to the body

The bacterium in your mouth poses a threat not only to its surroundings, but to your overall health. Also, medications sometimes team up with these bacteria because they act in a way that reduces the saliva in your mouth. The reduction in saliva is harmful for you as well, because saliva acts in a protective way by diluting the acids and making your mouth toxin free.

Severe gum diseases also plays role in creating circumstances for diabetes and AIDS by reducing the overall level of resistance of your body. Let's have a look at a few other linkages one by one:

- Endocarditis. Endocarditis is an infection of the inner lining of your heart. The flow of bacteria from the mouth to the bloodstreams acts as a transportation towards this problem.

- Pregnancy and birth. Periodontal, a severe gum disease, has been linked with premature birth and low birth weight.

- Osteoporosis. Osteoporosis is a disease that causes bones to become weak and brittle. This disease is linked with periodontal bone loss and tooth loss.

- Diabetes. Diabetes lowers the body's resistance to infection by putting the gums at risk. Gum disease appears to be more frequent and severe among people who have diabetes. The relation between diabetes and mouth problems is the strongest of all the linkages. The inflammation starting in the mouth takes away the ability of the body to control the blood sugar levels. People with diabetes have a problem with the processing of sugar because of a lack of insulin, which is the very hormone in your body that has the task of the conversion of sugar into energy. Gum disease and periodontal further stresses up the issue of diabetes because the inflammation takes away the ability of the body to utilize the insulin properly. Diabetes and periodontal have a two way relationship as high blood sugar levels in the body make it ideal for the infection to grow. So the medication for both has to be used simultaneously as one triggers and worsens the other.

- Cardiovascular disease. According to research, heart disease, clogged arteries, and stroke are linked to the inflammation and infections that oral bacteria can create. The reasons are not that lucid, but both of these problems go hand in hand. According to statistics, up to 91% of patients with heart diseases have periodontal issues as compared to 61% of people with no heart diseases. The risk factors of both of these problems also appear to have common grounds. These include factors such as smoking, unhealthy diet, and excessive weight. While some researchers also suspect that gum diseases have a direct role in raising the risk for heart problems, the basic theory behind this research is that inflammation in the mouth leads to inflammation in your blood vessels. Now inflamed blood vessels are a bad sign as they allow less amounts of blood to travel between the heart and the rest of the body and as the area squeezes up the blood pressure rises. The fatty plaque can also break off the wall of a blood vessel and travel to the heart of the brain creating circumstances for a stroke. Another reason is that bacteria in the plaque, when teeth decay or get injured, can gain entry into the blood and can end up resting on heart valves, resulting in a condition called endocarditis.

3.3 Benefits for the mouth

Apart from the facts that oil pulling gives you whiter teeth and a cleaner bacteria free mouth, it also acts as a remedy for bleeding gums and rescues you from bad breath. It is also a treatment for dry lips and soreness of the jaws. But, the benefits as we generally described to you above do not stop at the mouth.

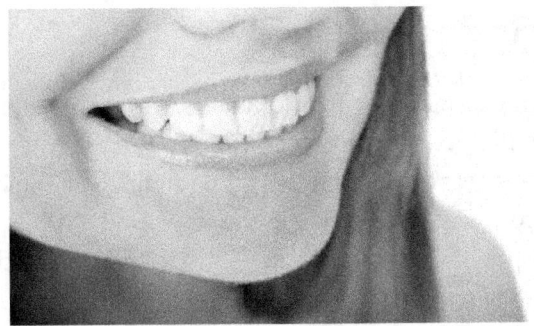

3.4 Benefits to other regions

- Headaches

- Bronchitis

- Chronic blood disorders

- Stomach ulcers

- Neurological diseases

- Liver problems

- Restricts growth of cancer

- Correcting hormonal imbalance

- Reduces inflammation of arthritis

- Helps support normal kidney functions

- Reduces risk of sinusitis

- Helps in coming out of a hangover

- Detoxifies the body from harmful metals taken from food and other sources

3.5 Scientific evidence on claims

Sesame oil contains high amounts of antioxidants sesamol, sesamolin, and sesamin along with a high concentration of vitamin E and fatty acids. What these antioxidants do is scavenger damaging free radicals in the body, absorb the negative forms of cholesterol in the liver, and aid it in its functioning. Several studies have shown the antibacterial capacities of sesame oil and thus they recommend that they reduce gingivitis and dental cavities. This was tested in 2007 when a study done on oral soft and hard tissues underwent a reduction in gingivitis after a forty five day use of sunflower oil. Similarly a study on the count of bacteria shows a 10% - 33.4% reduction in bacteria counts in forty days of oil pulling.

Chapter 4: Oil as a Supporting Actor

According to Dr. Sanda Moldovan, oil pulling is not magic, but your mouth is magic. When your mouth is properly working, it is the gateway to your entire health system. What oil pulling does is ensures the cleanliness of your mouth. It doesn't matter what type of oil you use as the result is the same; sesame oil is cheaper and can be used by the masses. As oil pulling helps in reducing the bacteria present in your mouth, it readily helps in reducing gingivitis and countless other health issues, as we'll mention later.

What seems dramatic to people has simple explanations in linking oral health to the betterment of the rest of the body. People with bad oral hygiene have a higher incidence for cardiovascular issues like heart attacks and strokes. Pregnant women with gum disease have lower birth-weight babies. The mouth is also connected to the sinuses and the ear canal; therefore, it leads to a decrease in these problems if kept clean. So everything is connected to the mouth and when we see it getting cleaned by the oil pulling we give it more credit and associate that to the betterment of the body, but are effective nonetheless as a supporting character. A cleaner mouth not only helps you in getting that refreshed feeling inside, but the reflection of the benefits shine on the outside as well. Being free from the problems inside, we can focus more on the other aspects. It also boosts our mood and you feel energetic.

Now an important matter is that you can oil pull regularly, there is no harm in being regular in performing this task but you cannot make that your substitute for brushing your teeth. Brushing also performs the important task of cleansing our mouth; its relevance cannot be ignored and should not be ignored. Yes, you may use oil pulling as an alternative to mouth rinse. Oil only goes about a millimeter deep so more serious infections and gum diseases do require medical attention and medications, otherwise you can cause some serious damage to your teeth. Oil pulling, in this case, is not the cure, but it can reduce the inflammation and discourage further bacteria activity.

4.1 Expert's advice

For every remedy that is naturally derived, people hold some sort of skepticism about it. It's not a strange idea, because since we are not aware of the technicality of the procedure, we tend to remain uncertain about it. The best solution therefore lies with the advice from the wise. Those people who have spent their lives in studies of the questions we are filled with, and they can surely come up with explanations to our doubts.

In this section we plan to guide you with the words of Chicago cosmetic dentist, Dr. Jessica T. Emery, who is the founder and owner of sugar fix dental loft. Reading the point of view of a doctor gives us more hope in the treatment and makes us truly believe what the procedure is worth.

According to her, oil pulling is an excellent supplemental therapy, but as we insisted earlier as well, she claims that it should not replace proper dental visits, as oil pulling cannot reverse the effects of tooth decay.

She insists that the longer the swishing process the better for the mouth, as more toxins can be absorbed and she gives twenty minutes as a rough estimate. Agreement on the alleviation of halitosis, reduction of gingivitis and cleaner and fresher teeth, and mouth breath is made by Dr. Jessica. Though she claims that she cannot prove every claim that people have witnessed or experienced, as an oral expert she can safely insist that since the basic troublesome part is the bacteria, its removal gives way for betterment in many aspects and prevention of decay is a prime example.

What basically happens is that most microorganisms in our mouth consist of a single cell. These cells are covered with a fatty membrane which is the skin of a cell. When we do oil pulling we use sesame or coconut oil, both of which have fatty acids, and when they come into contact with those microorganisms they stick to each other and are thus spilled out of our mouth. Coconut oil is preferred as half of its fat is comprised of a bacteria whooping ingredient, lauric acid.

4.2 Systemic effects

When bad bacteria enter the body through our bloodstream, they can get lodged in the wrong places, like scar tissue on the heart, thus making you very ill. Bacterial infection is one of the most common causes of endocarditis, and these initiate when germs from the blood stream enter our heart. Patients who have artificial joints, mitral valve prolapsed, or major surgery, need to be pre-medicated before dental treatment, because during the treatment bacteria can enter out bloodstreams. The more inflamed the tissues become the more the bacteria and the blood can travel to the heart creating problems for you.

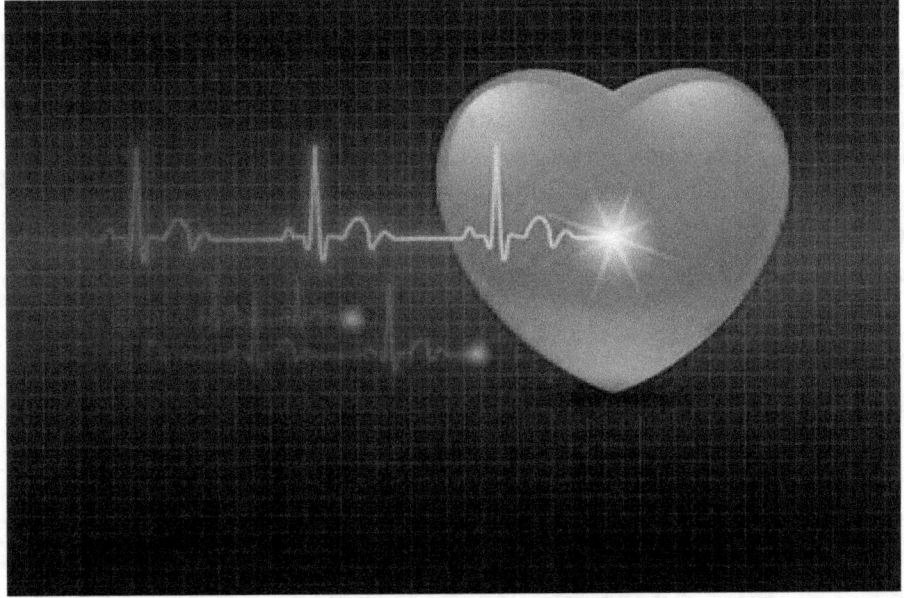

Pregnant women have a greater tendency to develop gingivitis because of the presence of hormones. The bad bacteria that enter into your body can also lead to premature delivery, in this case. Hence, oral health leads to systematic health being kept in check properly. All medical specialists advise pregnant women to be regular in their dental visits so they can avoid the problems like premature delivery or giving birth to low weight babies.

Systematically, oral health is related to many strong evidences of disease that can be really troublesome for you. So once it has been established that the ecology of the mouth is a crucial stronghold for the rest of your body, taking care of it becomes absolutely necessary for you. Oil pulling is a great way to make sure you keep the ecology healthy. It is better than mouthwashes since there are not various chemicals involved and that a pure and clean substance is being used for the safety of your mouth.

Oil pulling will not take your problems away in a single session and you have to be patient with it and give it ample time. Longer term benefits have to be kept in focus and it will only be of aid if we adopt this as a routine activity. The problem only left in legitimizing oil puling for the masses is that not enough clinical trials have been made to assure the people of the linkages that oil pulling may have to your system. However, it only has positive effects for everyone. Who wouldn't need better health care and whiter teeth?

Chapter 5: Multiple Options

Let's have a look at the various choices of oil that we may choose and their assorted benefits.

Sesame oil

Sesame oil is the one that is most recommended out of all the various options that we are going to present you with. Sesame oil helps in clearing out bad breath and gum and mouth disease. Let's have a look at the list of the other benefits sesame oil brings to the table.

- Heart feels better

- Depression is cleared

- Vision improves

- Underarm odor vanishes

- Helps in de-addiction

- Decreasing of pimples

- It moisturizes skin

- Cures dry or cracked heels

- Prevents hair fall

- Clears away sinus

- Complexion seems better

- Prevents allergies

- As skin gets better you look younger

- Digestion improves

- Back pain gets better

- Wrinkles disappears

- Cures insomnia

- Lessens dark circles around the eyes

- Removes hangover

- Stops weight loss

- Cure diarrhea

- Reduces pain in joints

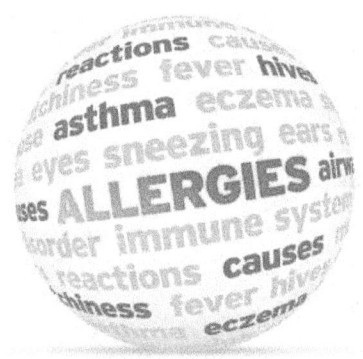

Sunflower oil

- Gets rid of gum and teeth problems

- Sensitivity condition is corrected

- Blood cholesterol profile is kept in check

- Wake up feeling fresh

- Hair gets thicker

- Reduction in lymph nodes swelling

- Increase in energy levels

- Blood circulation gets better

- Cravings decline

- Lungs do not feel congested and your breathing becomes more clear

- Cold sores decline

- Removes hangover

- Reduces fatigue

- Body aches get better

- Remove itch in ears

- Clearer vision

- Gases and indigestion problems cured

- Good for cracked heels

- Dark circles eliminator

Olive oil

- Mouth health improved

- Sinus cleared

- Nails grow fast

- Hair become thicker

- More energetic with mental clarity

- No coughing

- Softer hair and skin

- Eyes don't feel itchy or dry

- De-addiction from tobacco & alcohol

- Reduces back pain

- Nasal and ear blockage gets cleared

- Pores on face become smaller

- Brain fog cured

Coconut oil

- Appetite suppressed and weight loss

- Nerve pains are diminished

- Relaxant

- Reduces snoring

- Easy and clear breathing

- Heightened sense of taste

- Clears inner ear infections

- Moisturizes skin

- Increased agility

Cod liver oil

Cod liver oil provides us with the benefits of a glowing better skin and reduces our teeth issues.

Avocado oil

Avocado oil makes hair healthy and shinier, the bags under the eyes get flattened and the ever going issue of sinus gets cleared.

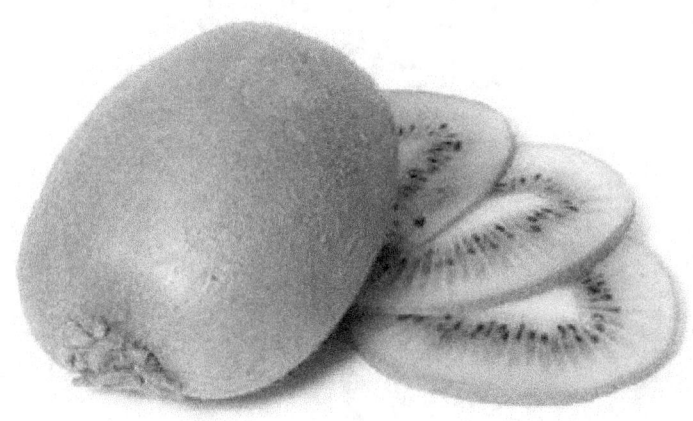

Cedar oil

Whiter teeth are the provision of this crucial cedar oil.

Canola oil

Better mouth health is the key advantage of canola oil.

Walnut oil

Walnut oil helps us in getting rid of gum problems.

Castor oil

Castor oil helps us in relaxing and induces sleep.

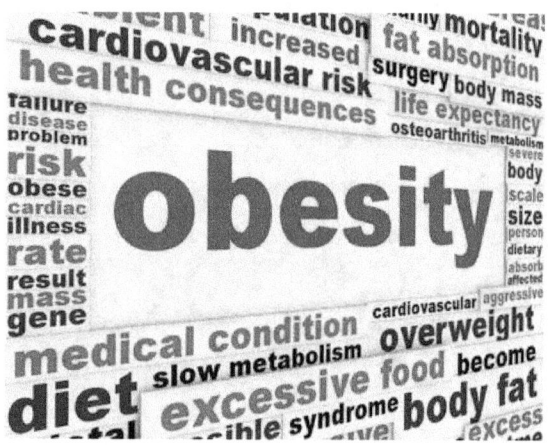

Black cumin seed oil

Drained mucus is the troublesome scenario from which black cumin seed oil rescues us.

Safflower

- Pulling sensation in the arms disappear

- Mouth issues resolved

- Reduces obesity and assists in weight loss.

- Becoming energetic and active

- Cures chocolate addiction

- Reduces scars

- Voice is improved

- Hair removal declines

Conclusion

You have read it all and understood it, hopefully. Believed some and shook your head at various parts, but there is one thing you cannot deny and that is the importance of a healthy mouth and the various impacts that it can have on our health system. All in all, oil pulling is a win-win situation for you. Look, cleanliness is important and we have strictly maintained throughout the course of the book that oil pulling is not a substitute to brushing teeth or paying regular visits to the dentist. What we have presented you with is an extra weapon that you can use to battle the germs entering your mouth. Yes it may replace your mouthwash as it certainly takes care of that particular task, especially having the prowess of whitening our teeth and taking our breath away (the bad one). Ultimately I find oil pulling to be a useful ancient remedy that we all will benefit from if we are regular in practicing it. It is not a medication that will bring side effects into the picture so there is no thinking twice before its adoption.

Author Bio

Muhammad Usman is a distinguished medical graduate of Allama iqbal medical college (AIMC). He is a professional writer who has been in the field for more than 4 years. During this time he has produced 10,000+ articles, blogs and eBooks on various niches related to diseases, health, fitness, nutrition and well-being. He is a regular contributor to several journals related to medicine and surgery. He is the editor of several journals and newspapers.

Check out some of the other JD-Biz Publishing books

Gardening Series on Amazon

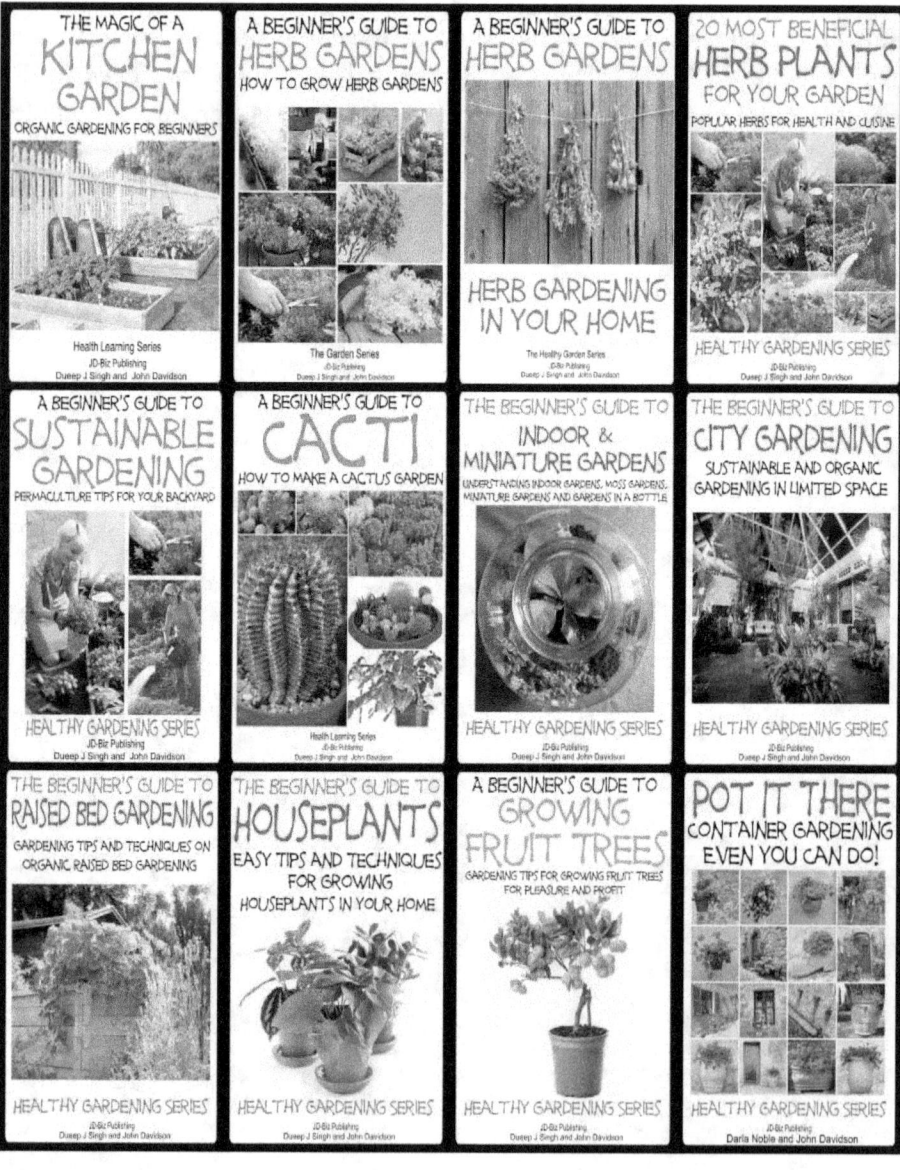

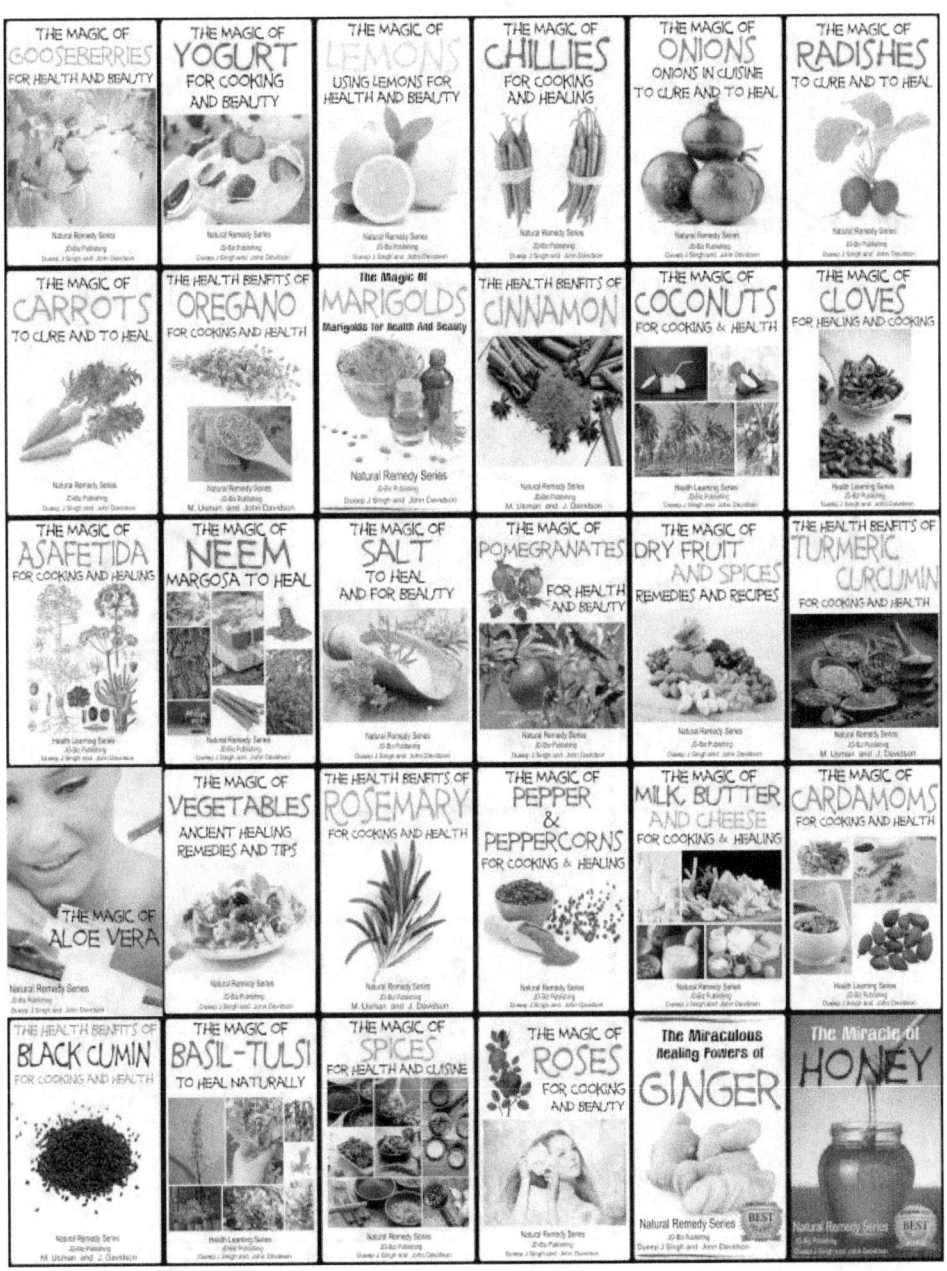

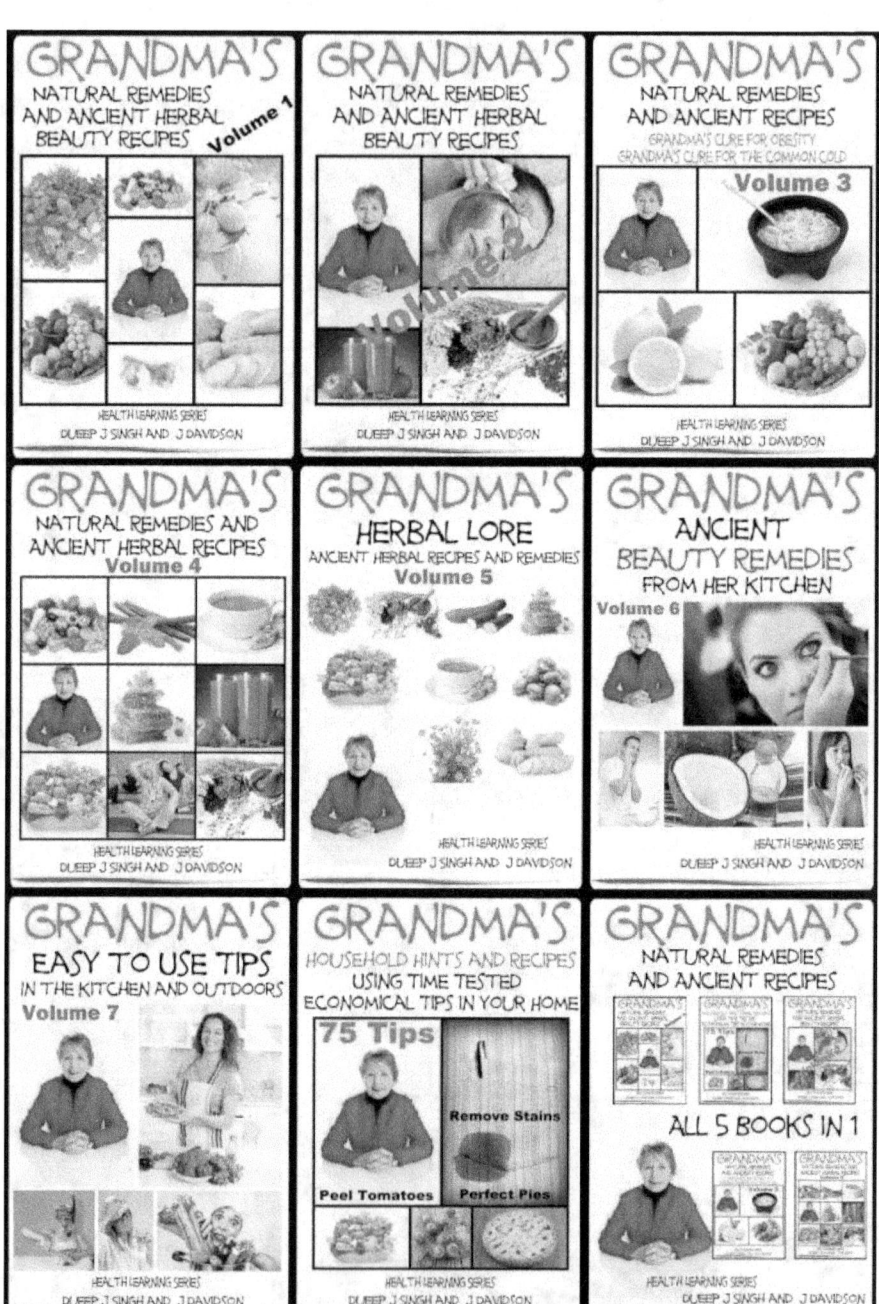

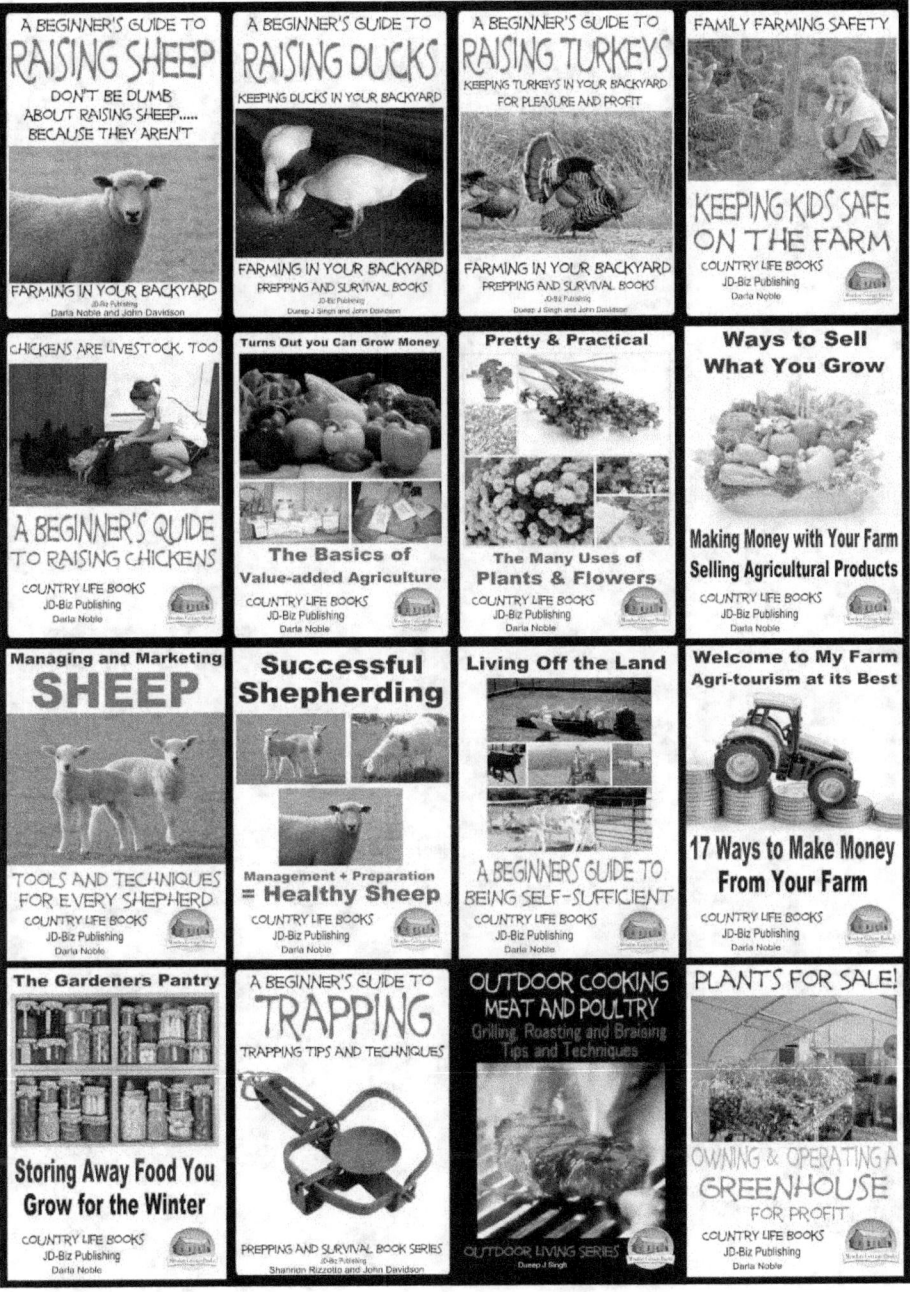

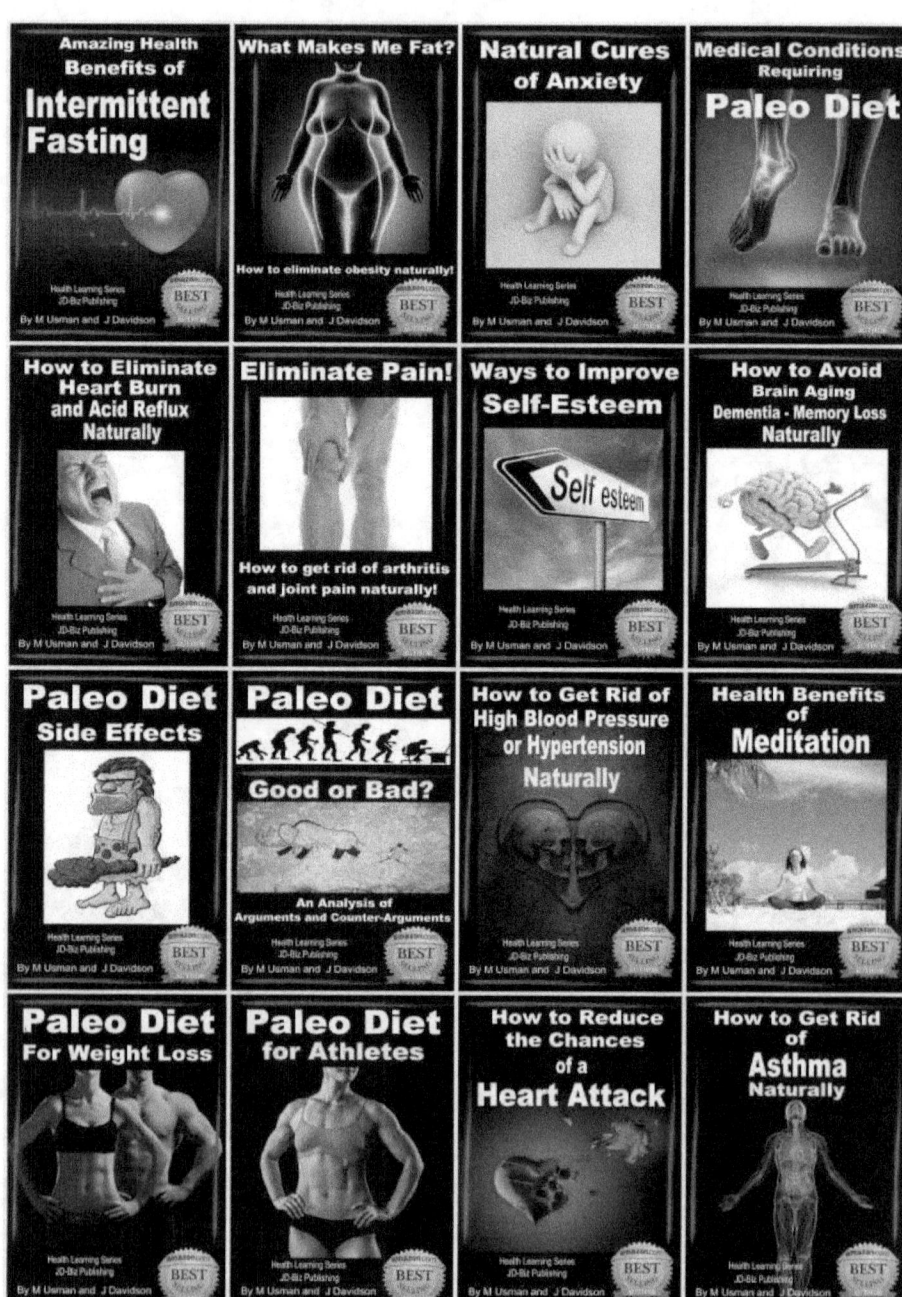

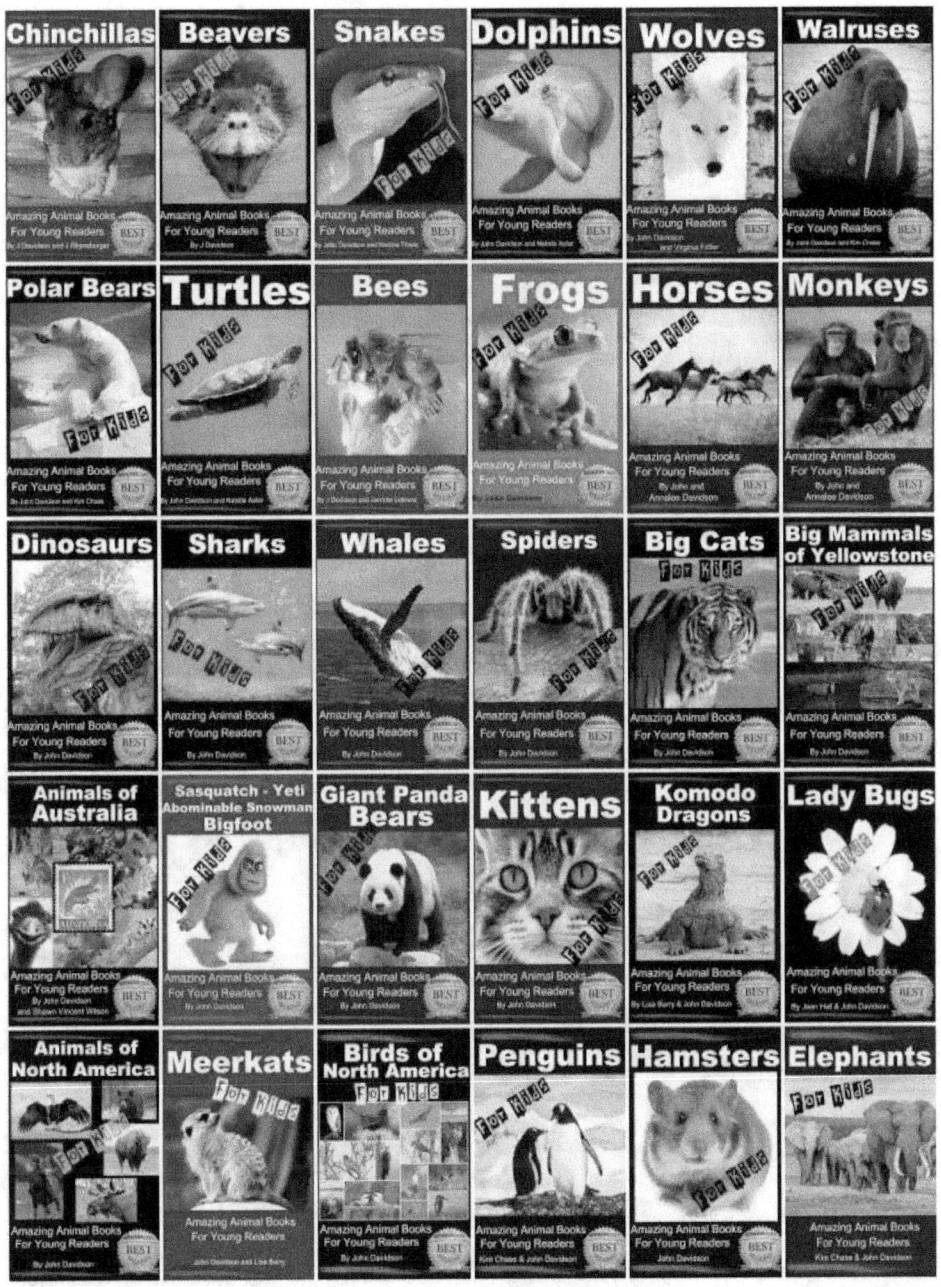

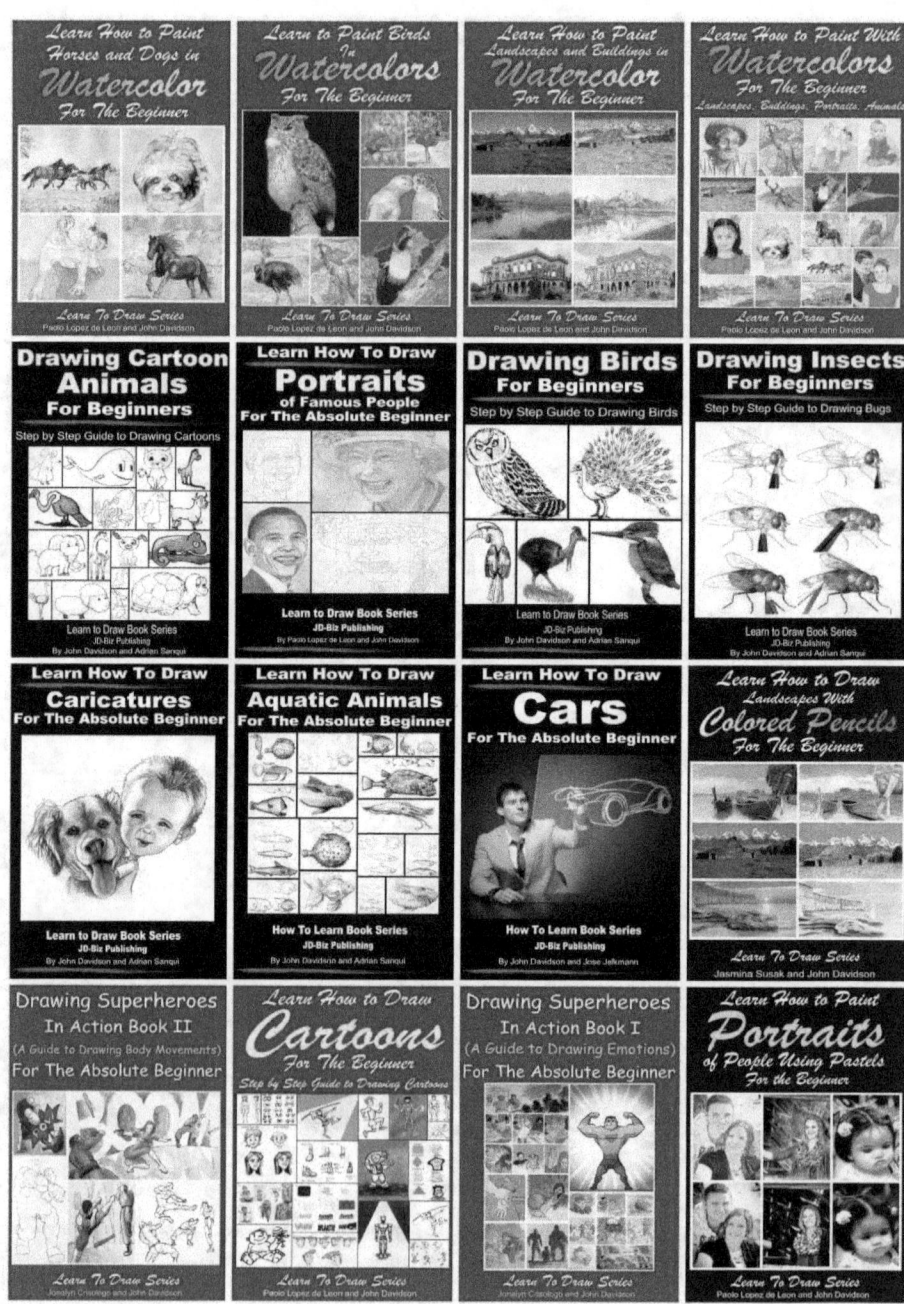

How to Build and Plan Books

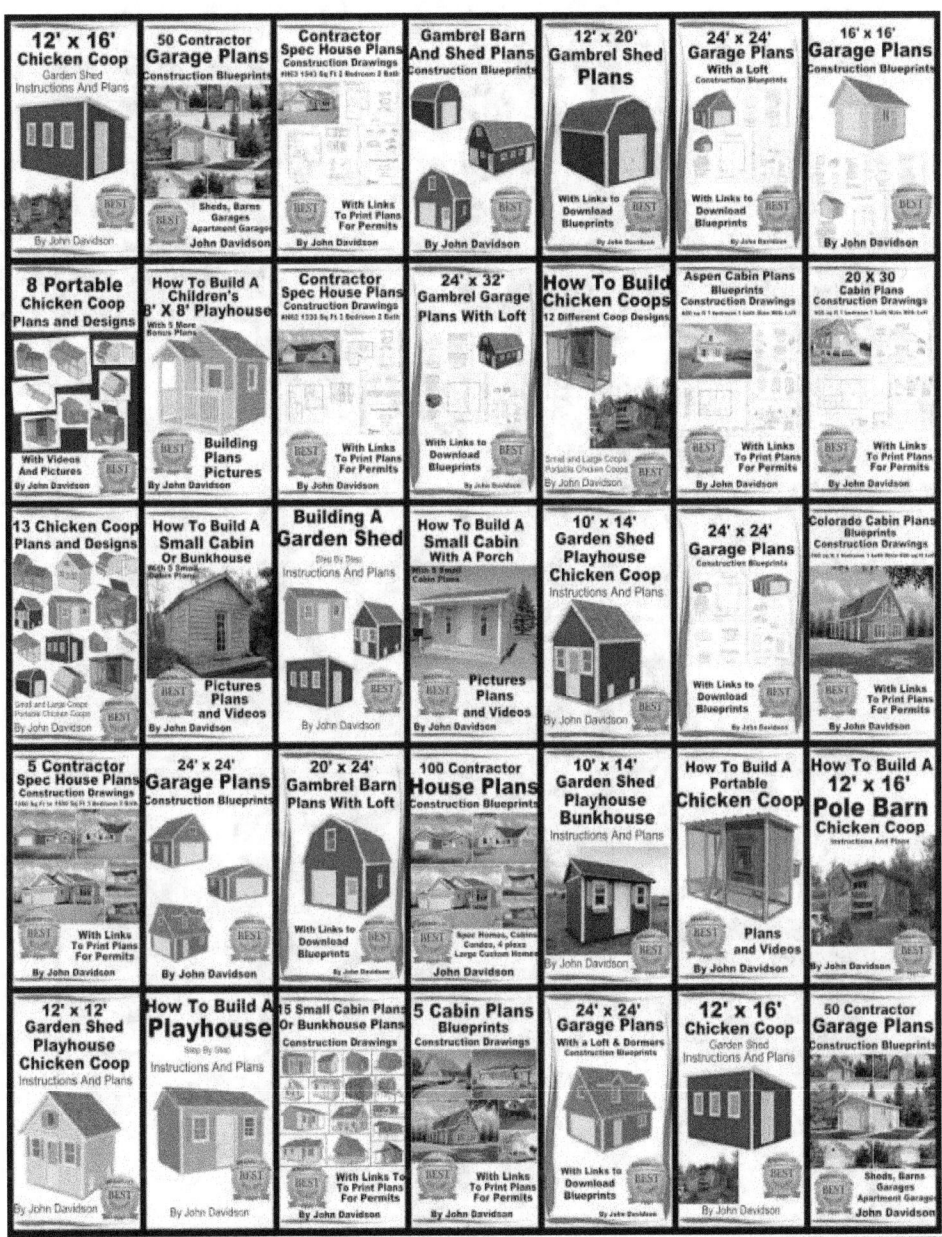

Entrepreneur Book Series

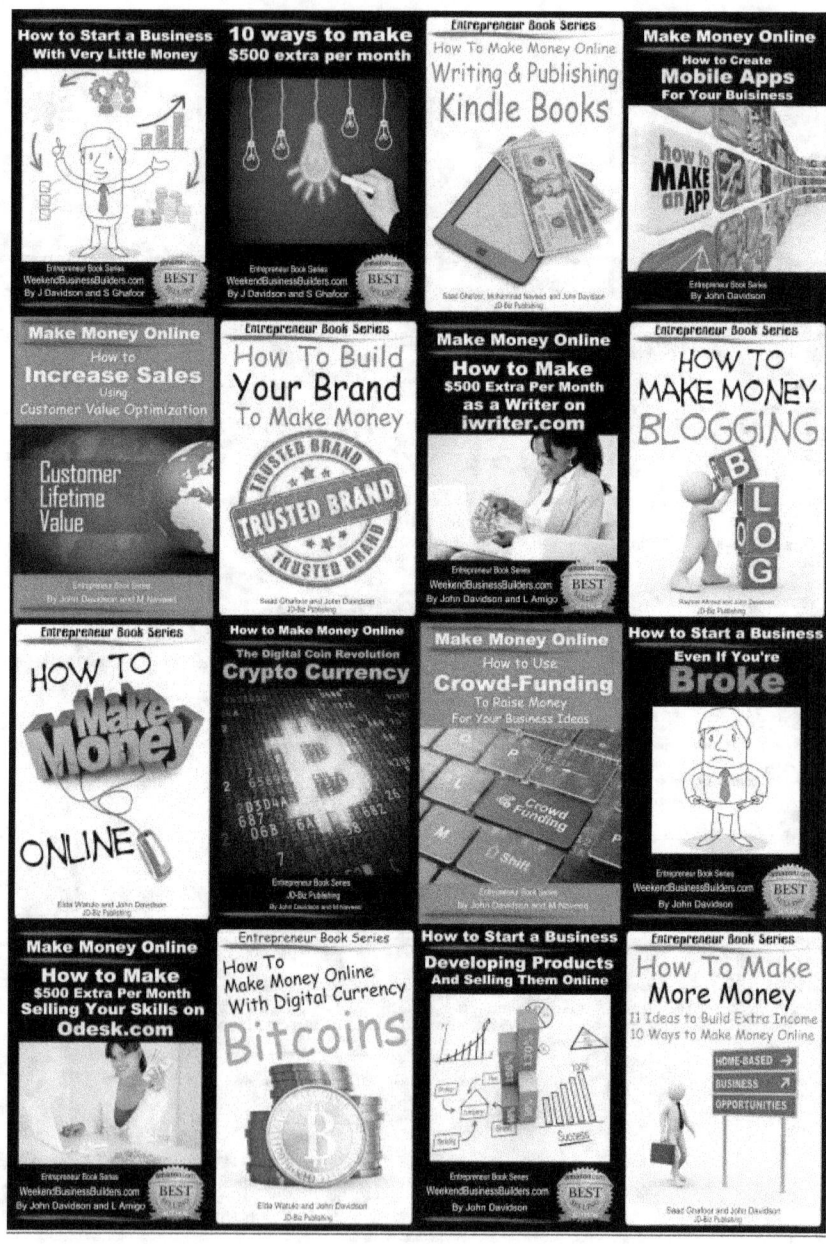

Our books are available at

1. Amazon.com

2. Barnes and Noble

3. Itunes

4. Kobo

5. Smashwords

6. Google Play Books

Publisher

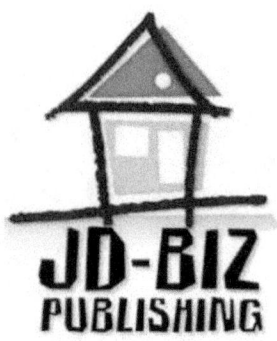

JD-Biz Corp

P O Box 374

Mendon, Utah 84325

http://www.jd-biz.com/

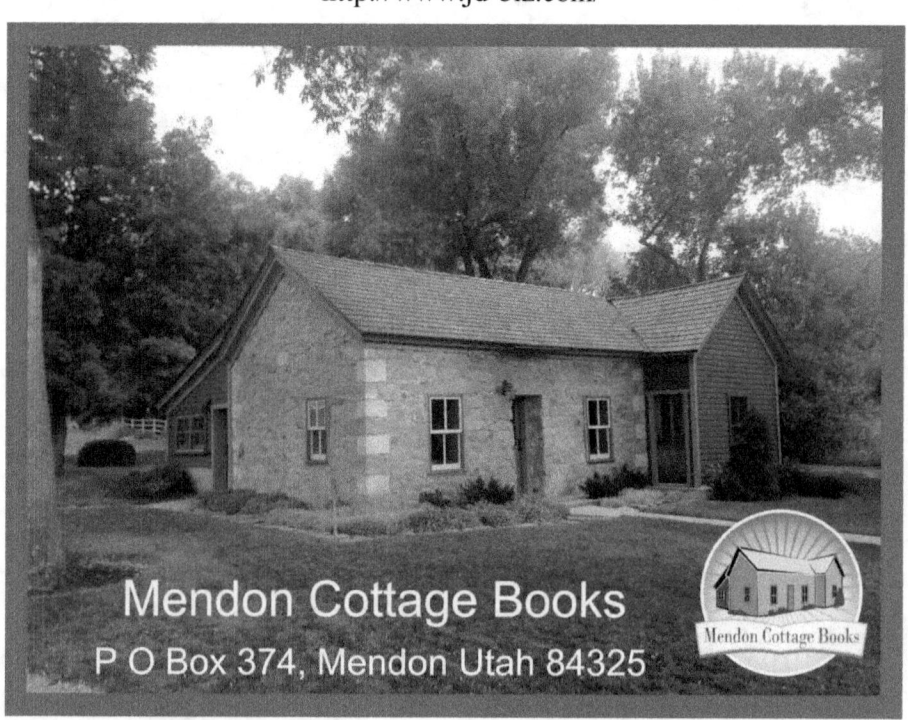

Mendon Cottage Books

P O Box 374, Mendon Utah 84325

www.ingramcontent.com/pod-product-compliance
Lightning Source LLC
Chambersburg PA
CBHW061928280526
45787CB00004B/1528